Dedicati

This book is dedicated to my mum, Margaret. She died two years ago. She was 86 and was suffering from Alzheimer's disease. Despite years of experience in nursing people who had this condition and supporting their families, as a relative myself, I wasn't fully prepared for the total devastation it can cause.

Heart breaking decisions had to be made, as mums memory failed. She fought us with every ounce of her stubborn strength but in the end she became unsafe. Funnily enough, when she moved into a care home she became happier, (most of the time)!

I feel a connection with other people who have lived through a similar experience and survived.

My therapy now is about trying to help others. Alzheimer's research is the future but sadly, the charity currently stands at 11 in the Yougov list. Cancer and children's charities are most popular and therefore benefit from greater funding. However, Alzheimer's disease will affect more of us, either directly or indirectly, than any other condition.

The proceeds from this book, will be donated to Alzheimer's Research. Thank you for buying my book and for supporting such a worthy charity.

Introduction

2020 and 2021 were, indeed are, extremely different years, mainly because of the impact of Covid-19, which has forced us to change our daily habits and our expectations. I have always thought that there wouldn't be another world war but a virus or natural event would be the thing that would cause devastation in the world as we know it. That this is just natures' way.

So it was that I found myself with holes in my day for the first time in my adult life. Having survived two lockdowns, the third began January 5th 2021. Struggling to keep myself busy, as the winter weather hampered my outdoor activities, I set about writing my book.

As each chapter and the people's stories came to me, I became consumed and couldn't wait to write the next paragraph. Although the original idea was to share my nursing memoirs, I soon realised that my focus was less on my experience of caregiving and more about the individuals and their lives. My interest in people has always been there, but during the process of writing this book it has become strikingly apparent to me that it is the connection with others and the intimate aspect of human interaction that I truly value. It's taken me most of my life to see that.

Contents

Community nursing in a nutshell

Community nursing is a role which is evident throughout history. Women became very skilled in treating members of their community. They often played the part of midwife too. These kind women, were unpaid but were totally dedicated to caring for others and this bought the respect of local residents.

District Nursing, as a profession began in 1887 when the Queens Nursing Institute was established. This charity, funded by Queen Victoria, developed a comprehensive highly skilled service to meet the needs of millions of people.

Some of the older District Nursing Sisters that I worked with early in my career, told me how their role initially, combined Midwife, Community Nurse and Health Visitor. Wow! A few even rode their bike to visit patients. They had to load all of their kit, (including bandages, instruments, birth packs for example), on the back, cycling a good twenty plus miles a day. They were on call day and night too. What amazingly strong women. In remote villages, the nurse was given a house to live in by the NHS, they couldn't have had much of a social life.

One District Nursing Sister, Molly, who I loved working with, had five children and she had worked most of their pre-school years. She managed by taking them to work with her, dropping the children off at various houses in the village, where kind women minded them. I had the pleasure of meeting some of these women and they recalled each child with fondness.

On certain days of the week Molly teamed up to assist the local doctor in outlying village surgeries. No appointments were made, people just turned up and waited in turn. On one occasion, someone was waiting to speak with the doctor to request a home visit for an elderly female relative. When Molly and the doctor arrived at the house, they found a body on the kitchen table with a sheet covering it. She was stone dead and had been there for four days!

In my role as a community nurse, I really enjoyed caring for palliative or chronically ill and dying patients. Visiting the person, as well as their loved ones, in their own home, was such a privilege. I certainly never judged a person by the type of house they lived in, or their belongings. For me it was all about the people and their pets.

One particular person and his wife I remember, lived in a huge mansion on a scale similar to a National Trust property but it had become a burden to heat and maintain. As their health declined, they lived in only four rooms. I've learned over the years, that it really doesn't make much difference how wealthy you are at the end of life, because the moment of death, like birth, is something we all go through.

My other specialty and passion, was leg ulcer management. Many of my colleagues despised them because they can be a challenge to heal and often involved a degree of noxious odour!

A great tip a colleague gave me when I first worked in the community, for assessing a patient, is to imagine you are a scanner. Starting at the head, working right down to the feet, checking for all manner of things such as facial expressions, breathing, body posture, signs of discomfort. My senses told me a huge amount. I think it also showed how I was engaged with them and focused down on their needs.

Back in the 80's, 90's and 00's we seemed to have more time to spend on each person, striving for continuity of care. As years went by, things changed, resulting in a reduced level of patient care. Managers gradually became more interested in the 'business' of health care, with computerisation a priority. Also, assessments for every risk you can imagine became the norm in what was an era of increased litigation.

I enjoyed my career very much and have many funny, moving memories (with an occasional odd one), from my encounters with patients. The recollections that follow, are just a few of them. They are in no particular order, all names are changed but they are all true to the best of my memory. It's my hope, that some of these stories will make the reader laugh and possibly cry, but also understand how truly wonderful and inspiring people can be in whatever health situation they find themselves.

****

Number 1

How excited was I to be working on the community? I'd chatted to the District Nursing Sisters through my previous job as a Marie Curie Nurse and we had got to know each other well. One day, I received a random phone call from them, enquiring if I'd like to work alternate weekends as a community nurse? Oh happy days! Family friendly hours and good money, what was there not to like?

No interview as such, just an informal meet and greet to run through the nitty gritty, kit, uniform and call device (bleep). I'd be called on the Friday evening, before my weekend, with my list of patients and all the relevant information. It amazes me now, to think I'd never done this type of work before and yet here I was, completely on my own, jumping straight in to the deep end.

It was with a degree of intrepidation but also overriding joy, I visited my first ever patient on the district - Chrissy. She lived alone, was totally blind and had a fiercely independent character. A type one diabetic she needed insulin injections morning and night, to maintain her blood sugar. Back then, we used glass syringes and reusable needles, which, after use, were rinsed thoroughly and put to soak in a sterilisation tank. How times have changed.

It is possible Chrissy was warned about my inexperience. Visualising her cottage, she directed me to locating all of the equipment I needed.

Chrissy lives on in my memory because she was an exceptional lady, so clever and funny and really kind. We'd share many giggles while I put the kettle on and made her breakfast. This was deemed our job as timing of injection with food was essential to prevent ill effects. With an acute sense of hearing, she could tell what I was doing and she'd point me to the cupboard for the item I was searching for.

Stories from her childhood and younger days when she had sight were clearly perceived as if they happened yesterday. Sadly, I can't recall them all but I do remember that her childhood had been restricted quite considerably after she contracted tuberculosis. Chrissy had to stay home from school for a year. I think that this experience early on in her life, taught her how to make the best of things and to be grateful. From then on, she threw everything at life, studying hard and working long hours for a pittance. What a woman!

I adored her attitude and positivity. Some people really teach us life lessons and she certainly did. I think I'm gifted with the ability to empathise with people, putting myself where they are. Just imagining her day to day existence with considerable restrictions and limitations, puzzled me. How does a person exist without being able to do basic things like reading, watching TV or to go for a walk? How do you maintain a happy demeanour? Watching and listening to her, I realised it was her routine and finding joy in the little things. Like the robin who came to sing it's beautiful song every morning that kept her going. She never failed to thank everyone who helped her, to show her gratitude. How could you not love her?

It's always astonished me, how some people suffer greatly through no fault of their own and yet appear completely unaffected. Good health is something that is often taken for granted. It's not until you haven't got it that this courage and strength comes through. Chrissy was a tiny frail lady but she had the mental strength of a giant.

****

Jack's story

A referral to the District Nurse team could come in from anywhere; a Social Worker, a neighbour, literally anywhere, but most were from the GP often a scribbled and illegible note in the District Nurse book. Our office in the surgery, meant we worked really closely. One such referral, described a gentleman with a new diagnosis of lung cancer, needing our support and advice.

The wind was blowing up a storm on the first day that I visited the patient. I introduced the District Nurse Service and how we could help, giving contact numbers, just in case. Well that's the basics, I was really there to 'suss' this gentleman and his family to get an idea of how they were coping with the diagnosis and eventually, the reality of death.

Mary, his wife was angry. Actually, that's an understatement. For an hour she vented all her feelings. The GP was next to useless, the NHS hopeless and to top it all Jack is giving up without even trying. "Stubborn through and through" was Mary's opinion on Jack's refusal of treatment. "Never thinks of anyone but himself!" Hmm! I took things slowly and listened to both separately.

Jack and Mary had always had a love/hate relationship. It was clear that Mary wore the trousers. Dominating, ruling the roost, worrying and moaning with only a rare glimpse of happiness. But in there was a rare sense of humour, very dry, sarcastic and at times black. For all the negativity that came out of this woman's mouth, deep down, there was also a fun loving lady at the core. If you got her on the subject of politics, she was away. A Labour supporter for life but having her beliefs challenged with the Blair government. When Mary offloaded her views on the state of the country, it was almost like a stress valve opening and the steam pouring out. Now Jack was under her feet all day, life had become unbearable. Unable to do anything, in her eyes, he was as good as useless.

Mary had a work ethic to make most of us cringe. Coming from a rural family in Yorkshire, life had always been hard. School ended at 14 going straight into piece work in the local factory. At 18, she joined the land army which she fondly recalled, having made friends for life. A chance meeting and dance at the local pub began a romance and they were married before she knew it. It was Mary's only shot at relationships, so she had to get on with it. Their lives became, like many in the post war years of bearing children and learning to bear each other! And to top it all, Mary had to help Jacks parents, as their health deteriorated.

Fiercely independent and struggling to make ends meet, she took in clothes to mend and alter, just to add a few shillings to the pot. It's hard to imagine the reality of their lives at that time. Husband working all hours god sends and when at home, he was probably asleep. She was bringing up the children and working every spare moment.

Jack was a man of few words. A man who had never caused a fuss or a scene, just got on with life in an orderly way. Making his living from gardening and the land, he didn't need to do that much interaction with humans. To him it was perfect.

When you got Jack on the subject of the land or the seasons, his smile went from ear to ear. Jobs that are always done at certain times of the year, and never in all his working years, had he ever changed this routine. A man of precision, some might say obsessional, but once taught, he could not change.

With the dawn chorus, Jack started the day, although now, not a necessity, but a habit. He told me how he would make haste to get outdoors and the first chores underway, always happy to be up and working hard.

As Jack became confined to his chair and the oxygen cylinder, his whole world changed. No more outside, no more freedom, no more interactions with nature and feeling the cold air on his face. For the first time, he had to communicate with the wife throughout the day!

Both Jack and Mary were intriguing and I struck up a bond with each almost instantly, but in quite different ways. Honesty and reliability was my focus with Jack, no beating around the bush. If he developed a problem, he promised he would call me. That was the deal and I promised that I would work on it but might not be able to sort it completely. Mary needed a lot more support, essentially to start the grieving process and at the early stage, her needs were greatest.

Grief is a weird emotional event for some people and it's not unusual to show itself as anger. Mary clearly loved Jack, not in a lovey-dovey way, it was much deeper than that. They were like a see-saw, opposites but in balance and dependent on each other. Understanding this, when Mary was firing negative criticism towards Jack, was important because it wasn't meant. In fact, it was the complete opposite.

Over about six months, I visited every two weeks or more if needed. The slow deterioration in Jack's condition was evident, by visible weight loss, and increased breathlessness. We had a way of talking about his psychological needs and what he understood about what was happening in his body.

Foreign travel was something that Jack had always wanted to do but never got round to. So we decided that when he died, it would be a wonderful trip to a beautiful place. We were on the same wavelength and we had many laughs on the banter around this concept. It is possible to be cheerful in these times. If humour helps then why not?

When he decided the destination, I knew that he believed that he was beginning the dying process. Flights booked, was another step closer.

Bags packed but still laughing, through extreme shortness of breath. Jack was controlling everything and I could see that he was enjoying it. As he slipped more and more in to unconsciousness, I kept the banter going, telling him his flight was ready to go and his luggage was on board. On the final day, I told him he had been in the departure lounge for a while and that he could take off anytime he liked. I knew that he could hear me. A squeeze of my hand and he was off.

Mary surprised me. In the final week, her approach to Jack became softly sympathetic and her hard exterior dissolved. She had reached a point of acceptance of Jack's situation, she relaxed and she enjoyed sitting with him, holding his hand.

Palliative and terminal care can be beautiful and for me in caring for both of them, I felt a huge sense of joy, achieving a good end to Jacks life and their seventy-year relationship.

Mary soon went back to her usual self, moaning about the state of the world. That was how I knew she was alright!

****

The cat lady

Sometimes a referral is made to the District Nurse team on behalf of the person in their best interests. Carers were involved with a lovely older lady, called Iris. Her incontinence was increasingly difficult to manage, which not only became a health issue for Iris but also a health and safety problem for the Carers.

I need to describe the back story to this lady. Iris had been an only child, to older than average parents. Intelligent and bright, she had won a place at university, which was unusual for women then. Sadly, before she completed her degree, she had to return home to help care for her parents, whose health had deteriorated but also, she had to leave the man who she had hoped to marry.

In a blink, life for Iris suddenly changed from scholar to carer. She disliked it intensely, but felt it was her duty. They all lived in a big house with beautiful gardens. The natural world and her pet cats became her escape. Dedication to her parents, meant no opportunities for her own relationships and so she thought of her cats as her loves.

Over years of caring, Iris became more reclusive from the outside world. Her neighbours were never considered, she disliked people, preferring her animals, who were loyal and understanding. Totally engrossed in literature and music, living a private life, without any modern conveniences.

Inevitably, the house deteriorated, vermin moved in and eventually it became uninhabitable, although Iris disagreed. After lengthy negotiations, Social Services put a caravan at the bottom of the garden for her to live in. A strong, almost selfish attitude, meant it was very difficult to help her. Iris believed that she was entitled to ignore everyone and all advice. Social Services had drawn up a legal agreement with her prior to moving, to enable the Carers to work effectively and safely.

When the district nurse team were called in, the caravan was in a state. Iris refused to wear incontinence pads, despite the carers best efforts. Chair cushions and bedding became soiled and the smell of ammonia, stung our eyes. Discarded, wet pads littered the floor because to her, she didn't need them. Even the floor was beginning to bend in places from the constant pools of urine, so we walked very carefully, for fear of falling through!

Fleas become another problem. Iris still loved her cats dearly but they had now multiplied and they became unmanageable. During our visits we would see fleas jumping everywhere but Iris insisted that we were making it up! A conspiracy to have her cats taken away. She hated us, indeed anyone who told her the truth.

An animal charity agreed to intervene to treat the cats, which Iris had had to accept or the cats would have been removed on the grounds of neglect. Sadly, some had to be euthanized for humane reasons.

People like Iris are thankfully now few and far between. However, when you do come across them they are usually 'characters', quite stubborn, often funny and quirky. Most people who require nursing care are concordant with health professional's suggestions because it makes sense and it's in their best interests. The patients who present challenges, are the ones that give the greatest reward and personal satisfaction.

Over a long hot summer, we continued to visit Iris because her health was declining. On opening the caravan door one day, the smell hit us full on. We took a deep breath and entered. Iris refused to open any windows so the combination of heat and smell became intolerable and we were forced to keep stepping outside to breathe. Social Services were called, to arrange a multi professional meeting, including a mental health assessment. The whole environment became too much on many levels but health and safety was top of the list.

After much discussion and persuasion, Iris was invited to spend a few days at a local nursing home. The selling point, was that the home had a small selection of cute fluffy animals for residents to pet. Also Iris could take her cat.

None of us believed that she would stay, however the opposite happened and she didn't want to leave. Every morning she went down to see the animals and her face was a picture. Almost instantly, her health improved and she relaxed into a new routine. No more fighting, angst or worry, all that was behind her and we breathed a huge sigh of relief. Our job was done at last.

Although it was tough to care for Iris, it was also a pleasure because she was a lovely lady. There's usually a reason for a behaviour, a bit like a child who misbehaves if they have experienced abuse. In lots of ways, Iris had suffered when she was younger, through sacrificing her ambition and potential. I liked to chat to her sometimes about which flowers were out and the sweet birdsong. We shared a love of all things natural. So many memories of her make me smile.

****

Compulsive Care

Everything seemed normal at first. A dedicated, very caring son, John was looking after his elderly mother Louise. He had given up work and moved into the same house as her. As her health and mobility declined, he asked for help to manage things like incontinence and mobility.

Louise was a very quiet, softly spoken lady. It was quite difficult to assess her without being interrupted by John. Her facial expressions were telling me that she wasn't happy but she seemed too afraid to elaborate. Over a few weeks, it became clear what was going on. John was caring almost too much.

During one visit, we noticed stacks of yellow waste bags laying around the bedroom floor. Also, Louise's skin around her bottom and groin, was extremely red and sore. John had been informed about the way the incontinence pads worked, in that changes were required a maximum of three times a day (unless soiled by pooh). Skin washing also usually twice a day. It turned out that John was changing and washing, indeed scrubbing his mother, every hour.

In all my days I'd never seen anything like it, especially from a man. Not stereotyping here, but it's usually a woman who takes the care role in a family. It was impossible to talk it through with John because he just didn't want to hear us. To him, he was doing a good job, however to Louise, it was a kind of abuse.

As a team we were very concerned and took the appropriate steps to protect Louise. You'd like to think that someone in senior management would have jumped into action? This was around 1996 and systems were not always as we'd like them to be. And so it went on.

John became more obsessive around outside germs coming into the house. He never went out. Shopping was delivered to the door whereby John washed every item. All door handles were covered with cling film and anything we touched was binned.

For our own safety and for witness purposes, we visited in pairs. From the moment we arrived he was watching us and telling us to don protective equipment. It was rather unsettling but we tried to work with him in order to help Louise.

Community nurse training does not cover mental health and I'll be the first to admit that we were seriously out of our depth. All nurses are taught about the 'duty of care' which basically means, to do no harm or neglect a person who is in need. This concept is usually quite easy to apply but when serious mental health issues occur in a care situation, it proves complicated.

As with most conditions, things gradually got worse. John believed we were out to get him. I discovered that he was taking a cassette recording of all our interactions without our permission. There were stacks of cassette boxes everywhere.

Anxiety and stress took its toll on John in the end. He clearly wasn't sleeping, he lost weight and neglected himself. Communications between us became almost impossible because he frequently lost his temper and shouted at us.

Louise's health declined after several months of this care and she was admitted to hospital, never to return home. I think she gave up. We never found out what happened to John.

It's an experience I never want to repeat. To be honest, it's much less likely to happen nowadays anyway, as all forms of abuse are recognised and acted upon much earlier, thank goodness.

To be fair to managers at that time, knowledge and information on unusual types of abuse, wasn't as readily available as it is now. However, they were naive and only listened to one side of the debate, which was John's.

Every time we discussed our issues we were made to feel we were exaggerating things. We were not supported at all by our line managers. Our District Nurses though were brilliant and as a team, we became very close. It is possible to laugh through hard times and we drank a lot of wine too!

****

Cuckoo!

Our very funny and dry humoured GP, wrote the new referral which, he added was, 'a special one, just for me'! I had a great working relationship with him. He knew, I was passionate about palliative care.

The house, let's say politely, hadn't seen a paint brush in at least 30 years. We found Delia downstairs, laying on a bed by the window. She had terminal breast cancer which was fungating, (ulcerating through the skin, similar to a cauliflower). She had refused all treatment 'thank you very much' claiming that she did not need any help.

You could say that Delia was in denial about her condition but she really wasn't. Convinced that everything was fine and she could manage herself, repeatedly exclaiming that she didn't know what all the fuss was about.

Edward, her middle aged son, lived upstairs and had very little to do with his mum. If he was younger, he would probably have been diagnosed with dyslexia or another similar learning disorder. He couldn't keep eye contact and avoided all communication with anyone. We were pretty sure he had no idea what was going on with his mother.

So I'll paint the scene. Every surface that surrounded Delia was covered with piles of old letters and junk mail. Probably ten years' worth at least. Then there was the snarly little she devil of a dog, called Layla. This dog was small but had a mouth full of razor sharp teeth. Every time we tried to wade through the detritus and get close enough to Delia to assess her wound, Layla appeared, growling and barking with teeth bared ready to attack.

Fortunately, I had a ready supply of dog treats and we had a cunning plan! We attempted to lure the beast out, by dropping treats along the tiny gap from the bed to the back door, where upon a moderately encouraging 'kick' to the backside of said animal, ensured we could actually do our job safely. Dear Layla, was completely ruined by Delia, even being fed from her plate, so there was no way she was going to give a toss about our requests.

This worked for a while but then Layla grew wise to our devious ways. The GP suggested a permanent solution - buy a piece of fresh meat from the butchers, stand on the opposite side of the busy main road, open the front door and call for Layla. So helpful!

Cuckoo, was the word Delia called to summon you close and to give out her orders. She lay in bed like Cleopatra and with a click of her fingers in the air, she repeatedly called 'cuckoo, cuckoo'! We all found it exquisitely funny, however also slightly demeaning. 'Tea with two sugars' she'd bellow (no please or thank you), and if it wasn't exactly right, she would not drink it. We got to know exactly how her servants felt back in the day. Later, she told us about her childhood, which made it more understandable.

A child of quite wealthy parents, distantly related to royalty, she was used to a life where servants waited on her hand foot and finger. As a child, she mixed with cousins and relatives from the Bowes-Lyon side of the royal family. On the wall hung a large fine oil portrait of five young girls, one being Delia. The others shall remain nameless.

She would love to tell stories from her younger days as a journalist, interested in the fight for women's rights. Living in post war London, a single care free girl, who enjoyed the high life and wild parties for the adventurous! Even we had a few raised eyebrows. Many of these tales, seemed to be on a similar theme to the Profumo scandal and around the same time. There weren't many dull visits with the delightful Delia.

Two children of different fathers (she suggested) and no man to support her, I think life was quite tough for Delia, although, I believe she managed some financial agreements with the absent (married) men. Never one to complain, she made the best of things. I believe both boys enjoyed a private education.

To our credit, with bloody hard work, we won her over in the end. Our whole team had a soft spot for her, despite her behaviour's which nearly sent *us* CUCKOO!

With most people in this state, things can only get worse, as weight loss and weakness increase. Mobility for toilet purposes was essential obviously and the mass of tumbling litter in her room proved a disaster waiting to happen. Delia barked her orders at us, refusing to let anyone interfere with her documents as there were "letters of great importance" within the stacks! Negotiations around this issue ensued and she relented to allow us to bag some up but under no circumstances must they be thrown away.

One day, we found Delia asleep on our arrival. A, (my colleague) and I went for it. Twenty or so black bags were speedily filled and placed in the spare room. Delia went bonkers when she woke, accusing us of stealing her personal items. People in the street outside could hear her screaming obscenities at us.

Eventually, she ran out of steam. We felt awful but we had to do it. Over and over, we apologised and tried to explain why we did what we did.

Edward, upstairs, quietly minding his own business, was clearly used to his mother's extreme behaviour and didn't enquire as to what the problem was. We felt obliged to give him the reasons for our actions and the mass of bagged rubbish in the dining room.

While we had his attention, we tried to warn him of his mother's deteriorating condition and of what to expect in the weeks ahead. He showed no emotion at all. It was as if he hadn't heard me and as soon as he could, scurried off upstairs again.

Upon entering the house one morning, I found Delia laying on the floor. She'd fallen in the night and had a suspected broken hip. In the ambulance she gave us the royal wave and 'bye bye darlings' in true Delia fashion. I could see she was distracted by the rather handsome paramedic attending to her needs.

In the office later, we all gathered to give each other a good pat on the back for a job well done. We never saw Delia again sadly. I believe a friend took the lovely Layla and Edward still lives in the same house in the same conditions.

As a human being Delia was a great lady to know. Her personal history was so interesting and different to the lifestyles of most people of her generation. Having a journalist training, she had the ability to recall factual stories about real events. But it was her hilarious narrative and upper 'classiness' that combined into great entertainment. She was special in many ways, a sensitive caring animal lover, resilient and tough but also stubborn as hell.

****

Legs, legs and more legs!

In addition to palliative care my other forte was leg ulcer management. For most nurses, leg ulcers are not popular because they often present with odour (that's putting it mildly) and they can be difficult to heal, frequently taking months and years. But that's why I liked them - for the challenge. During my degree, I studied leg ulcer care, so I became skilled and quite knowledgeable on the subject. My family understand that I am obsessed with legs, it's very sad. Both of my kids grew up used to seeing medical journals, with full colour pictures of pretty gruesome wounds, laying about everywhere. They are scarred (excuse the pun), for life.

Research from the 1990's made fundamental changes to leg ulcer care in the UK, which was then rolled out nationally. Previously, patients received variable care, according to their individual nurses' experience and this resulted in poor healing rates. I remember many patients used to wash their own bandages for several uses, to save the NHS money. It's inconceivable in today's health care arena.

Compression bandaging was and still is, I believe, the most effective way of healing leg ulcers. A risky treatment, if applied too tightly, can cause the circulation of blood to the feet to be compromised and further, to gangrene. Nurses had to understand the physics of this treatment in order to get the compression just right - tight enough but also, not too loose either.

Over the years I've treated hundreds if not thousands of people, most in leg ulcer clinics. Out of these, a few remain in my head for unusual reasons, which I will endeavour to explain.

****

Help!

Spinster sisters, Sybil and Elsie were an old fashioned pair who ran their lives as of the times of the 1950's. Elsie was housebound, so we visited on a weekly basis to bandage her leg, which had a large ulcer. It was not unusual for them to get quite stressed about things going on around them. Visits could take a while, mainly to reassure them and to convince Elsie that the treatment was working, albeit slowly.

It was summer and the weather was quite hot. Our day was coming to an end thankfully but then the phone rang. Unable to understand the reason for the call, I tried to calm the lady down. She was hysterical, panicking, and desperate for help. After encouraging deep breathing, I ascertained it was Elsie, it was her leg.

Upon arrival, Sybil ushered me in quickly. She was in a state too. There, before me, I saw hundreds of maggots wriggling their way across the floor from Elsie's bandaged foot. Sybil was deployed to hold Elsie's hand and calm her breathing, basically to distract her, while I dealt with the other end.

Maggots or larvae are sometimes used as a form of treatment for cleaning wounds but they are produced under sterile conditions in the lab. However, these were opportunistic maggots, caused by a fly creeping up inside the bandaging and laying eggs. The combination of hot weather and odour had been irresistible for said fly. Elsie's reaction was totally understandable, but in actual fact, it wasn't too bad. My challenge came when I removed all the bandages whereby a multitude of maggots made a run for it, in every direction. Swiftly, Elsie put her leg in a bucket of warm water which helped relieve her anxiety while I tried to catch the maggots.

The situation was farcical. I tried to make it look like I had control but I didn't. As fast as they were put in a rubbish bag, they were escaping. After half an hour, we started to relax but then out of the corner of my eye, I spotted one creeping out from under the chair. What would normally be a thirty minute visit took ninety. I was exhausted and as soon as I got home, I felt compelled to strip and shower immediately!

On the plus side, the leg ulcer looked beautiful and clean and I'm sure the maggots aided the healing process. It took a long time for Sybil and Elsie to see the funny side of that afternoon's happenings.

Ben

In one of the UK's most innovative and advanced leg ulcer services, I gained valuable knowledge and experience but also, the people attending were from a larger age range.

One of the youngest was Ben, an intravenous drug user and addict of many years. He was so desperate to find a viable vein, that he would apply a tourniquet to his thigh and inject at various sites below his knee. This caused vein engorgement and permanent damage, which then caused a large venous leg ulcer.

Ben was given the usual assessment and following a full explanation about the risks, compression bandaging. He agreed that he wouldn't touch his bandages whilst at home and if he had any issues would call us immediately.

We didn't hear from him, so assumed everything was ok. At the next appointment, it was clear that everything was not ok. Such was Ben's need to inject into his leg, he'd cut the bandages away above and below the ulcer leaving a tight band of roughly 6 inches in the middle of his calf. Tissues above and below swelled and the band tightened further.

Ben had inadvertently severely reduced his circulation to his foot and lower leg. There are only a handful of times in my career that I've had to dial 999 but this was a medical emergency.

About ten days later, we found out that Ben had had to have an above knee amputation. Sadly, he died from complications. We felt shocked and almost guilty that we hadn't considered what he might do to himself. Hindsight is a great thing but we all concluded that we were working in his best interests and our actions had all been correct.

****

A stonker!

In 2004, we decided to move to the south west. We found that many of the locals were wonderful, country people with lifestyles set in stone. I guess every area in the UK, has its own unique challenges when it comes to people's behaviour's and understanding. It's not about intelligence but more beliefs and culture.

S (another colleague), and I thought we were the A team in leg ulcer care. Nothing fazed us. We had enjoyed many experiences together but one chap floored us.

It involved a fifty something year old man, who I'll call Brian. He was nervous and uncomfortable to admit that he had a problem. For months, he had been trying to manage himself because he was working long days and simply couldn't spare the time. I think his personal hygiene and general appearance suffered, also through being so busy.

A rather potent smell wafted along the corridor to our room, Brian had arrived. It was beyond anything we'd ever dealt with before. S and I were on the verge of throwing up and took it in turns to discreetly leave the room, in order to gasp some air.

After plucking up the courage, we revealed the ulcer. It was the size of a dinner plate and bright green! Brian however, didn't appreciate how bad it was. We explained about compression bandaging, as his treatment, twice a week. Work was his priority and it was very hard for us to get him to agree to that. We bent over backwards to give him the last slot of the day, a time usually used for admin and clearing up.

You couldn't help but like Brian, for he was just a hopeless bloke in many ways. Our patience was well and truly tested sometimes though. He'd forget or turn up late for his appointments, making us late home, again.

Months later and a mega amount of effort from us, his ulcer was almost healed. Brian was going to Cornwall for a long weekend, to attend his daughter's wedding. We agreed to supply stockings, so that he could get his decent shoes on but also maintain the compression. Obviously, he was given detailed instructions and advice on how to manage them himself.

The following week he returned for his appointment. We nearly cried.

Brian had worn his stockings as advised but when he squeezed his foot into the smart slim fitting shoe, he had wrinkled and pushed the stocking back half way up his foot. This then cut into his flesh, like a rubber band, causing the circulation to stop. It must have been incredibly painful but he hadn't thought to get help.

Poor Brian had to go to hospital or risk losing his foot. About a year or so later, his ulcer and foot healed. It was such a relief and a huge achievement. Didn't we celebrate that one?

****

Dog encounters

Previous to this, I worked in a country practice in a beautiful rural area. Some leg ulcer patients were very well known to us, being regulars for years. Leg ulcers often recur quite regularly. No sooner are the patient's ulcers healed, then they're discharged but are then back again with an ulcer.

Robert was one such patient. A club foot and polio as a child had left him with numerous issues in his feet and legs. After a number of attempts at surgery to right the club foot, the surgeon gave up. All his life, he wore medical boots, specifically fitted to his foot shape with callipers to support his lower leg.

It was quite obvious that mobility was quite difficult for Robert but he was a determined man and extremely independent. Every time a medical problem popped up, he would find a way to manage it. We admired his spirit and did everything we could to support him.

When Robert told us he was going on holiday, we wanted to help him. This meant that he needed a change of bandages just before he left. I arranged to visit him at home.

I'd never been to the house before, as he had always attended the clinic. With bag in hand, I wandered down the garden path. All of a sudden a large black Labrador bounded up to meet me. Dogs have never been a problem for me, as they've always been a part of my family. However, I got a different feel to this furry friend. Barking and teeth on view, I knew what was coming.

Attack! My adrenaline must have kicked in because the next thing I knew, I'd somehow jumped the gate and got away. Phew! Robert followed up to check that I was alright and apologised repeatedly. Breathing deeply, I regained my composure.

Robert reassured me that dog was safely locked in a room and the coast was clear. I ventured in again. As I got near, the dog flew past Robert and sunk his teeth into my arm and then as I turned to run, took a chunk out of my tunic, very near to my bum! Again, I legged it to safety. Physically shaking, I sat down in my car for ten minutes. It transpired, that the dog had figured out how to open the door of the room where he had been 'safely' secured.

Third time lucky? I agreed to go back and redress Robert's leg because there really wasn't any other choice. He was desperate to go on holiday and his treatment couldn't be done any other time. With the dog controlled properly by the wife this time, on a lead in another room, I nervously entered. I'm a pretty fast worker but I've never done a job as quick as I did that day. A part of me was quite annoyed with Robert. I think he knew and felt sorry for his lack of foresight with a dog, who clearly was not friendly to strangers.

On arrival at the surgery, my colleagues spotted something was wrong. As soon as I stepped through the door I collapsed in a heap. The adrenaline had worn off and I was a blubbering wreck. Patched up, jabbed with a tetanus injection and a strong cup of sweet tea, it wasn't long before I was able to see the funny side.

You'd like to think I'd be allowed to limp home to recover? Oh no! One call left, a quick injection for a disabled lady and then home. My lovely, kind, caring colleagues (not) thought it would do me good to do an 'easy' visit.

Standing outside her house, I heard the loud bark of a dog. It was all too much. I froze. I shouted to her, with a slightly hysterical tone, that the dog had to be put away from me, or I wasn't coming in. I was terrified. Luckily, the lady obliged, but I felt dreadful. It wasn't her fault. Once she learned what had happened to me earlier that day, she sat me down with a cup of tea and gave me a huge hug. It had been quite a day.

An incident form had to be completed, with details of my actions. Surprisingly, it didn't look good on paper. My manager was quite annoyed with me (no change there!) for putting myself at risk. I suppose she was right. I got a severe ticking off. I probably wouldn't do it again but hindsight is a wonderful thing. I saw his needs above mine.

****

Sexual healing?

Chas where do I begin? My memories of this gentleman are numerous so I'll try and recall as many as possible. He really was unique and a real character but also, a bit of a social misfit, living a secluded life. He could recall dates with ease, such as on February 16th 1952, he had a consultation for a kidney infection. I am not exaggerating, his brain was like an enormous filing cabinet of facts and dates, as well as names.

A type two diabetic for years, he had developed many secondary conditions associated with this disease. Extremely poor vision, foot and leg ulcers, as well as kidney problems. Chas had a lot to contend with.

An ingenious inventor, to enable him to hear, (add deafness to the list), when someone was at the door, he balanced a string of empty cans on the inside door handle. As the handle was compressed, the cans dropped, clanging loudly on to the floor. Who needed modern door bells?

Chas had unusual tastes when it came to food combinations. One of his favourites was tinned sardines cooked in the microwave with whatever was floating (I kid you not), around his fridge, such as cauliflower, eggs, beans. Yuck!

We deliberately avoided visiting at meal times as the smell nearly wiped us out. On a few occasions, I made an excuse to leave the house to get something I'd conveniently 'forgotten' to bring in, just to breathe.

Feeling guilty, I admit once or twice that I delayed my visit, as I detected the most disgustingly foul smell emitting from his house. On days when you weren't feeling at your best, it could fill you with dread.

I think that I sound quite judgmental in writing down these memories specifically relating to Chas but it is just my way of relaying what we observed. He was quirky and we liked him for that.

His preferred dress style to his lower half, was a small towel wrapped around his waist, rather like a flappy miniskirt. No underwear, he liked to feel free! During his leg ulcer care, positioned kneeling on the floor in front of him, I looked up to talk to Chas, only that wasn't all I saw. Legs parted, his meat and two veg (on the large side), appeared before me. Blimey! It was unclear if Chas did it deliberately or not.

Community nurses generally, are a fairly unfazed breed. It became a challenge amongst us, of how to give his care without lifting our eyes. He was harmless enough to us but he had vocalised some sexual needs.

Nursing is like many other services, constantly changing according to the latest research. The nursing process, trending from America, was a means to assess the patient holistically, involving physical, psychological, social and sexual details. To be honest, most nurses would skip the sexual section, as it was quite difficult to ask questions without feeling awkward or embarrassed.

On the occasion I reassessed Chas, I had a student with me, so I thought I'd better do it 'properly'. How we kept a straight face I'll never know. Chas elaborated about his regular visits from a prostitute for sex. The funniest thing was his no nonsense factual way he told us. Of course I documented everything briefly and moved swiftly on.

My student and I looked at each other with raised eyebrows in the car after our visit and then we burst into fits of laughter. This experience made us chuckle for sure, but at the same time, Chas was entitled to enjoy himself, whichever way he chose. Good on him.

A few days passed. My colleague, J passed me the phone, the call was for me. It was Chas, enquiring if I was married OMG! I was gobsmacked. When I eventually found my voice and composure, I told him I certainly was not available. Raucous laughter could be heard way down the corridor, as was often the case in our team. J never did let me forget that.

Kidney and bladder problems increased gradually for Chas, which was partly managed with a urethral catheter (a long thin tube, inserted into the bladder, through the penis and a bag attached to the end to collect urine). He disliked it intensely and it caused him considerable discomfort.

During this time, we believed he was still sexually active, despite having a catheter. Numerous issues happened, somewhat inevitably, where we would be called out for a blockage or occasionally the catheter 'fell' out.

As a means of keeping Chas and us happy, (we were exasperated by the frequent call outs), he was fitted with a supra pubic catheter, (inserted into the bladder through the abdomen), thus leaving his penis free for his pleasures.

It was not unusual to find jugs of urine on his table, next to his already disgusting looking food. We tried to educate him about hygiene but Chas had to do it his way.

In fact, there were endless issues with his home safety and personal wellbeing, that were not ideal but we had to accept, that he had the right to live the way he wanted to. Unless someone is in danger of significantly harming themselves or others, there isn't a lot you can do. Although some days we found it hard to visit Chas, we never thought any less of him. He was a one off and experienced the world slightly differently, that's all.

****

Carer, or not?

Anna, a fifty something year old lady, lived with her husband Fred. Morbidly obese, Anna had huge problems to overcome just to live each day. Every kind of psychological help and support had been offered over a number of years and yet Anna just got bigger and bigger.

The front room of the house was converted into Anna's bedroom, as she could no longer manage the stairs. Toilet functions were done using an extra-large commode by the side of her bed. It was so sad to watch her struggle to lift each limb into position for standing and then become completely exhausted by the effort of walking a few steps.

Fred appeared to enjoy caring for Anna but seemed a little overly controlling at times. He almost enjoyed seeing his wife becoming more and more dependent on him. Meals were all prepared by Fred. He was responsible for providing temptation. It wasn't that he didn't know what he was doing, for he was and still is, a highly intelligent man.

Healthy eating plans, drawn up by dieticians, were advised for Fred to use in shopping and cooking. He acknowledged all of the information and pledged to try harder. Still Anna got heavier. Fred believed the weight gain was caused by a hormone imbalance because he had only been providing healthy meals.

In the end, Anna had a gastric band fitted, which is a procedure that reduces the capacity of the stomach, so after a small amount of food, the person feels full. Also, a liquid calorie controlled food substitute was prescribed for Anna to drink instead of eating.

Initially, the weight reduced and we were hopeful. However, Fred became overly obsessive about other parts of Anna's care, almost to the point of arguing over every detail, frequently threatening legal action. It became very uncomfortable to visit Anna because of Fred's behaviour. We had a duty of care to Anna, which we dutifully fulfilled, although relations with Fred were extremely difficult.

Anna's weight slowly increased again over a few months but we couldn't figure out why. Both Anna and Fred declared that she was only taking the liquid diet. In their view it was due to hormones.

At a multidisciplinary meeting, we discussed the possibility that Fred was not being truthful. All professionals who visited Anna observed and listened to their daily activities. The rubbish bin held clues to the typical foods eaten, whether by Fred or Anna. Fish and chip waste was the predominant choice and judging by the quantity, for more than one person. Numerous chocolate wrappers and cake boxes were also seen. Signs that solid foods had been blended to a liquid were evident in the dishes.

There is a recognised condition called Münchausen Syndrome By Proxy, where the carer is in fact the abuser. We had our suspicions that this was happening, but proving it was another matter, especially as he became more angry and unhelpful towards us.

As I mentioned previously, general nurse training does not cover such issues or how to handle them. To be fair to us, Anna's GP didn't have a clue either. Mental health services were not interested, for reasons of consent and personal choices. We had nowhere to turn, we knew about it, but couldn't stop it.

Sadly, Anna died in hospital from multi system failure I believe, which, maybe true. We will never know. Poor Anna always demonstrated a deep fondness for her husband and was very grateful for his care. I believe, that he probably controlled her psychologically from early on in their relationship, so it almost became normal.

On reflection, I guess Anna was happy living the way they did, albeit a short and difficult, restricted life.

I still see Fred around town occasionally, but I always avoid eye contact and step aside. My mind is sure of what I experienced back then and I will not change in that belief, although there is no proof or evidence.

****

Time warp

This story is set in a beautiful, rural location and a family home for generations. Desmond and Mary are brother and sister, never married, and have lived together since they were born. Hard work is all they've known, no luxuries or modern comforts. As they approached their late seventies, health issues were inevitably happening to both of them.

Following a referral from the GP, we were asked to assess Desmond's legs. A dirt track, with grass growing up the middle, was the main route in. It was winter and my tiny car groaned as I gingerly negotiated the craters and puddles.

Mary came out to greet us, shouting and accusing me of trespassing. She calmed down once she understood why I was calling. Mary was stone deaf so communication was not easy.

Inside the tiny little front door of the cottage, I perceived a strange feeling. It was dark and gloomy, musty, generally quite grim. To the left of the hearth, Desmond sat, silent, anxious. He avoided eye contact. I greeted him with a cheerful 'hello' and introduced myself. Silence.

I identified the cause of his problem immediately. His legs were positioned right in front of a roaring fire. The skin was red raw, blistering, swollen and leaking fluid all over the floor. A right mess.

After explaining the cause of his leg problems and how to effectively treat the wounds, I looked for a place to wash my hands. Mary waddled in with an old enamel bowl and placed it on the table. She then heaved a heavy black iron kettle to the bowl and filled it with hot water. A huge block of green soap and a clean towel was also supplied for my use. It was like I'd stepped into another world circa 1930.

Mary cooked all their meals on the fire, as there was no electricity supply. With no other form of heating, they huddled together to keep warm. It was one of the most old-fashioned houses I'd ever seen, both in practicalities and in their lifestyle and beliefs. Both Desmond and Mary lived their lives as their ancestors had, resisting change and modern developments, determined and stubborn.

Looking around the main living room, I saw an assortment of glass boxes, where stuffed animals posed in a country scene, frozen in time. My godfathers it was creepy. They could be seen as art I suppose, everyone to their own. Every time I visited, I had to mentally prepare myself for the imprisoned animal carcasses, as well as the monster spiders lurking in the corners waiting to pounce!

In a bedroom where Desmond was resting one day, I turned around and saw a huge mute swan standing in a box. Somehow I managed not to swear out loud! Call me hypersensitive, but I think if I'd seen it as a museum piece in an institutional setting, it wouldn't have shocked me quite as much.

It does beg the question, why on earth would you want to sleep in a room with a dead swan? Now't as queer as folk. Clearly hidden from visitors view, maybe it was an illegal killing? I don't know, but I couldn't get out of that room quick enough.

To the front of Desmond and Mary's cottage, was the route of a public footpath. They had protested and contested this path for years with the local council but to their disgust, they had been unsuccessful. They viewed walkers as trespassers and Desmond had threatened a few with his shot gun. Quite intent on scaring innocent people who were just following a route on a map, he purposely sent the message to the local community to steer clear or else. As a result, both Desmond and Mary were ostracised from their community, which left them alone with no friends. A very patient and kind nephew was their only support.

Sadly, there was no laughter with Desmond, indeed he barely spoke to us. He frequently removed his bandages believing that 'the air' was best! It was an exasperating situation and as a result of his non concordance, his legs became infected and deteriorated considerably. Hours of our time were spent explaining the treatment to Desmond but he refused to listen.

Eventually his symptoms required hospitalisation, much to his disgust. We didn't see Desmond again. I think he required further care in a home, leaving Mary alone up on the hill. I think I'm correct in stating that together with a kind solicitor, Mary succeeded in rerouting the footpath away from their land. I seem to remember a newspaper article about it. So 'good on you' Mary, wherever you are.

****

Eye, eye!

Through the years and years of visiting people in their homes I've rarely been offended by personal possessions. Yes, some have been peculiar but I view most people's tastes with humour. Indeed, the 'stuff' that surrounds a person, is fascinating to me, as it tells their stories. I am particularly interested in art and I often spent more than a few minutes admiring my patients' collections as a way of opening conversation.

Not long ago, I visited a man whose mother in law had died recently and her collection of giant dolls (each one about 4 foot tall) were being stored temporarily at his home. He was apologetic for the state of his living room. An already over cluttered space before the dolls moved in, they were crammed behind, on and between the furniture. I don't know how I contained my giggles.

From every angle, numerous blank faces with huge eyes were staring right at me, seemingly scrutinising my every move. It was like a scene from a horror movie, where the dolls suddenly activate to life with an evil intent! Each time I looked up, there they were (I'd clearly lost it at this point)! The only way to keep my nervous laughter from escaping was to turn my gaze down while seriously focusing on the task in hand. That took some doing.

What a bizarre thing to collect. I guess the mum in law had a childhood love of dolls that just grew (in more ways than one), with her. Apparently she was a powerful woman and gave strict instructions as to the future of these dolls following her death. My gentleman felt frightened that the mother in law would come back and haunt him if he didn't carry out her wishes. Bless him.

****

Adrian

As I've already mentioned, palliative care plays a large part in the daily work of community nurses. It's so interesting and a privilege to be involved in because each and every case is so different and individual. Sometimes people opt to stay in their home until the end and this last choice in life is always respected but can't always be achieved.

People who live alone for instance, have to accept that during the final stages of life, there will be long periods when they are on their own. Support and care services just can't cover 24 hours every day.

Another consideration is the home layout, particularly the space that there is for nurses and carers to work in. Extra equipment is often required for a number of reasons such as hoists and commodes for instance.

Adrian had been referred for palliative care. Off we went to assess him but a journey that should have taken ten minutes took forty. After many wrong turns and enquiries from local dog walkers, we found him, living in a field.

At the entrance to this little community was an assortment of decorations. The best description is 'out there'! It was like walking into a street in Glastonbury. Positioned each side of the entrance, a few temporary buildings colourfully bedecked with 'art' of every pattern and beast, gave us the feeling that we'd entered another world.

Three or four shop window manikins, fully dressed in all manner of colourful, shining outfits and hats, posed for the visitor.

We were soon spotted by a very helpful friendly guy and he directed us to the bottom the field. Parking the car, we walked down, dodging the dog pooh, observing many delightful creations along the way.

We should've expected something unusual. Adrian's home was a shepherds hut. It was tiny, probably 6 feet long and 5 feet wide. His bed ran width ways across the far end of the hut, he was curled up but apparently quite comfortable.

Trying very hard not to view this environment negatively, we assessed Adrian and took our time to get to know him. Fiercely independent and totally happy with his lot, he was adamant that he wanted to stay in his home till his dying day. It was not the right time to challenge his decision.

Often on our visits, we'd sit outside in all weather's, chatting, as it was too cramped in his hut and seating was minimal. Adrian's daughter tried to persuade him to go into care but he wasn't having any of it. I've met many people similar to Adrian in my time and the one thing that's certain is that no one is going to change their mindset.

Time eventually brings change, as the symptoms increase and with that a dawning realisation that the final stages of life might be easier if care is available through 24/7.

So after about three months, Adrian agreed to move into his next door neighbour's wooden chalet. It was a huge relief all round. He was completely comfortable for the first time in months, laying in a full size bed.

On good days, he still popped back to his hut just to sit a while. Being in control and still able to make choices, was all he wanted. Visitors joined him from his community, keeping him laughing and reminiscing. Many of these people valued him as their father figure - you could feel the love and respect that they had for him.

It's hard to relay the relaxed aura around him and in the whole community. You could sense a spiritual essence of peace and love, it was beautiful to experience.

When the end came it was awesome, if you can describe death that way. A quiet, dignified end to a life well lived. Job done.

Adrian's daughter, who supported him constantly, was extremely grateful to us, not only for respecting his choices but also for supporting her throughout his illness and for a few weeks after.

It's difficult to quantify the affect that is felt by family or friends when the end of life of the person they love comes. Some are literally terrified, anxious, worrying about every new problem that arises or hung up with guilt and regrets. Alternatively, but rarely, some are totally happy and relaxed with their situation.

Hours of listening, holding hands, reassuring, and supporting is required, sometimes for months. Inevitably, you get to really know these people. Invariably, more time is given to the family or friends than the patient.

Adrian had been a difficult father to love and care for and the arguments they'd had were recalled and relived frequently. All his daughter needed was an ear to download to (me), this enabled her to vent but also back off. It worked.

Living and working in the same area, I frequently bump into people around town, who were previously carers. We never forget the experience but I feel the connection through their smiling eyes. Sometimes the sight of me in the supermarket is enough to reduce them to tears! Maybe because I remind them of their loved one or it could be in response to my ugly face!

****

Ted

I have to include this amazing man's story for many reasons. Endurance, courage, resilience, humour and acceptance.

Face and neck tumours thankfully, are quite rare and in my forty years I've nursed about a dozen people with them. I rate them in my top five of worst conditions to get. The reasons are, I suppose, pretty obvious. Having said that, I'm talking about a good eight years or more ago and treatments since, have made symptoms easier to bear.

The carotid arteries and jugular veins serve the brain transporting blood up and down through the neck. Air exchanges happen through the airways, also positioned centrally and digestive processes begin in the mouth, so it's a hot area for essential systems to function. Tumours often grow in to neighbouring tissues, disrupting the function of these parts, which can lead to instantaneous death. More often the person suffers with a sore mouth, repeated infections, breathing difficulties and considerable pain. Put these together with facial disfigurement and the package of symptoms is awful both mentally and physically. Having these experiences, I know that I would choose voluntary euthanasia, if I ever had the misfortune to be in this position.

Back to Ted. His tumour was clearly visible on the right side of his face around the jaw line and it had fungated through into the inside of his cheek. Initially, Ted needed help to dress this weeping area because he found it increasingly difficult to manage himself. It wasn't easy for him to accept our help. He was so strong and very stubborn but he also made light of what he was going through.

Right from the start, he joked around, it was his coping mechanism, so we had no choice but to join in. If anyone had overheard our conversations, where we deliberately pulled his leg and he ours, or our sarcastic comments directed both ways, they would probably have judged us as rude and offensive. This was the way he wanted it.

It was one of those situations where we were like actors in a play. It was Teds play and he was the director. Absolutely no honesty or open discussions around his feelings or thoughts about his or his family's future, unless he wanted to. He was another one in 100% denial.

Some terminal illnesses hide their progression from the onlooker, leaving you wondering if the scan and blood results were correct. With Ted however, it was obvious, although he didn't register the changes when he looked at himself in the mirror. It started as a fifty pence size tumour but soon became a 10cm growth, oozing brown mucous fluid.

Eating was near impossible, so a feeding tube was inserted into Ted's stomach to provide all his nutrients and fluids. One day, chatting about what I'd been up to, I told him about the

delicious meal I'd cooked the night before.
What a plonker! I realised what I'd done
immediately and apologised over and over. I
can't repeat what he called me. I don't think I've
ever goofed as bad as that.

Following this, we'd joke about the
extraordinary 'meal' he was having through the
feeding tube, - roast beef, roast potatoes,
Yorkshire puddings for example, washed down
with a nice glass of red. Being unable to enjoy
good food was one of the hardest elements of
his illness but he overcame it with his usual
humour. He was a great cover up artist.

To start with, he would down play his pain,
saying he was ok when he clearly wasn't.
Fighting every step of the way, he tried to ignore

doctor's advice and manage things himself. It wasn't nice to watch him suffer. In the end he accepted a pain killing patch applied to his skin which was a game changer. He talked to me about what scared him - being drugged up and sleepy all the time. It freaked him out. And so it was a fine line between managing his pain, whilst not incurring drowsy after effects. Sounds easy? Pah!

Over a long period of time, you get to know the signs when something ain't right. Tactful, devious detective work, without direct questions enabled us to distinguish what really lay behind the jokes. Ted was good at fooling most people but it didn't work with us, much to his disgust. Ha ha!

As time ticked on, the tumour inhabited most of the side of his jaw and neck. Our challenge was to apply a dressing that was functional and stayed in place, while also being removable without incurring too much pain. It was a nightmare and a true test of our crafting skills.

Timing of visits was lined up with Teds pre-dressing medication to create an optimal window of maximum pain control. Thankfully, he would be happy with a mid-morning visit, enabling us to scurry around to the early fixed time visits first, while he had enough time to get up leisurely.

Ted had a high priority in our workload and we tried very hard to achieve his needs. This was a time of high demand for our service and it stretched us considerably. Two nurses would spend an hour or more with him every day and as things got worse, another visit was organised by the late shift.

My brief introduction to community nursing, touched on the changes that I've seen over three decades. Ted was a good example of the total nonsense of attempting to quantify or cost care, because his needs were so complex and numerous. I guess all services have to be managed but it's impossible to compartmentalise accurately, ticking the required boxes, to justify the time that is spent in a visit. For example, as Teds tumour grew, so his speech became more and more difficult. He simply could not be rushed. Every word took immense effort and understanding him was a challenge to put it mildly. Sensing his frustration and limited energy, we had to observe and listen intensively.

During this period, he had some down days, where he would be glad to end it all. Also, his wife often worked away from home, leaving him alone and frankly, very frightened, although he'd never admit it.

Having known Ted for quite a few months, I became 'professionally' very fond of him. It's not recommended I know, as you do not want to favour one patient over another, but I'm sure other nurses would admit a certain level of a 'relationship' in similar circumstances. Ted was someone who I admired and revered. If he needed help, I and the team would be there.

Always reluctant to call us out, it made us more than happy to go the extra mile.

Fragile and painfully thin, Ted gradually lost his ability to move around the home easily. We joked that he needed a couple of pints of cream down his tube to fatten him up. Forever mischievous and generally mucking about as if nothing was happening to him but we knew deep down he saw the end was in sight.

Ted put his house in order and organised his funeral, as if he was doing his online shopping, I'm sure he got a bargain arrangement! Finally, with everything sorted, he agreed to go into the local hospice. His wife was exhausted, both mentally and physically, from caring for him night and day for weeks and weeks. Although he wanted to stay at home to die, he knew that it just wasn't possible and accepted it without a fight.

We said our good byes through the touch of our hands, 'everything will be ok' we whispered and 'make sure you behave yourself' and 'get ready for the best party' then off he went.

Tears are close as I write this, all these years on from when Ted died. Memories of him stay with me, because of his amazing spirit and huge strength of will. He was blessed and in turn, he blessed us with the knowledge and beauty of a person who was, for me, beyond all others - a super, super star.

****

Spiritual tip

I have no views on religion personally but I do consider myself as spiritual. Nature is the thing I am most connected to, be that animals, trees, birds, whatever. Tuning my senses to my surroundings is when I feel most relaxed and calm. On a few occasions, I've encountered a real spiritual experience with other people as the following story, will describe.

Motor Neurone Disease (MND), another despicable disease. Symptoms vary for individuals but in general, it starts with a minor weakness or malfunction such as a fall or numbness or slurred speech. No two people present in the same way and the progression differs too. At present there is no cure and the poor unfortunate soul who gets it, has a limited future of slow, sometimes painful deterioration until death.

Richard was diagnosed with MND in his early sixties. A husband and father, full of energy and laughter and highly intelligent. Both he and Roxanne (his wife) had total disbelief of the diagnosis, their whole world changed in a moment. They were a couple who clearly loved each other deeply but who also could fight like cat and dog. Many of the visits we did in the early days, were to calm them down and support each one without taking sides. It's another great skill of the community nurse - marriage guidance!

Both of them were feeling extremely angry about what life had thrown at them and were scared stiff about their future. It was quite normal, arriving to find a full blown row in progress, which would continue around us. Roxanne frequently literally shook with rage and frustration. She suffered from a nervous disposition anyway but this almost caused her to have a nervous breakdown. So holding her together was our main goal because without her, he couldn't stay at home.

Richard passed his time by studying the horses and placing bets. He was very successful too, whooping with joy when the race was on and the 50 to 1 came in. He'd give us tips on the dead cert in the 3.30 at Epsom or whatever, but we didn't, for fear of the legalities of benefitting from a patient. The code of conduct for nurses is forever burnt into my brain. How annoying it was when said horse came in first!

A brilliant teacher, he taught us all the tricks about racing. The horses history, the jockeys weight and past winning record, the weather and the state of the course and the competition. My previous knowledge of racing was pretty basic, only winning a bet once in 1984, just after my daughter was born and the grand sum of a tenner! Richard enjoyed testing our knowledge, sometimes asking us to read up and then choose a horse. I'd deliberately choose a duffer because I liked the look of the horse or it had a funny name! He despaired at my hopeless ineptitude, but we laughed a lot.

Slowly, one by one, Richard lost his abilities. Simple things like drinking, chewing and swallowing food became unsafe because he would choke. With no other option except starvation, a gastric feeding tube was inserted and daily fluids and nutrients were pumped in directly to his stomach. It was a decision that later, caused lots of ethical dilemmas.

Speech, something we all take for granted, was stolen from his poor crippled body. After struggling with the basic communication tools on offer from the NHS, a speech therapist arranged for Richard to have a computerised voice system which he could operate himself. It made such a difference and it became a means for Richard to put his cheeky quips and filthy humour back into his world. We never failed to laugh in this house but we cried, some days too.

We watched as the essence of this amazing man, was taken away by a brutal, ferocious disease. He lost everything he loved to do, even down to the silliest things as being able to scratch his own nose or wipe his bum. Bearing all these losses came at a cost for both Richard and Roxanne. He suffered with severe depression and frustration. His brain was alert and active but his body was dying around him. Roxanne almost caved in, contemplating his transfer to a hospice because her nerves were in tatters. Somehow, she found the strength to keep going.

Discussion around death and dying, giving Richard respect to his choices about resuscitation status and where he wanted to be, helped us to achieve his wishes. He enjoyed planning his funeral and even wrote a eulogy. He wanted it to be happy rather than somber and tearful.

As with most MND sufferers, pneumonia is the thing that gets you in the end. Infection in the lungs from weakened muscles and not taking diet or fluids is nature's way and death occurs usually after a few days. Only for Richard, the feeding tube was complicating matters. Nutrition continued because morally and ethically we could not withdraw it. No one had thought to ask Richard to specify this, while he was able to. It became a horrendous problem, not only for him but for Roxanne and his son. Richard just couldn't die.

One weekend I spent every spare minute that I could with them. Richard had copious amounts of secretions in his lungs, he was literally drowning internally. To sit by his side and watch him fight for every breath, was awful and something you never forget. For his son, it became intolerable and he asked if it was possible to give him an overdose, (aka euthanasia). I've been in this situation before and of course, all I could do was support and reassure him, that it would come to an end soon. I kept hoping.

As another day dawned and he was still alive, Richard's son confessed that he intended to smother him with a pillow. WHAT? I was stunned into silence because I knew he meant it. Appearing calm on the surface while my mind was panicking about what I needed to say next, all I could do was hug him and let him cry it out. I'm quite empathetic, so I got where he was coming from. If I was in his shoes, I'd probably feel the same and this is how I started (don't panic, there's more). Like a duck paddling like crazy beneath the water but remaining calm and in control, I continued. I didn't want to reprimand him about the law and all that serious stuff, so I asked him to ponder two things. How would it make Roxanne feel? And how would he feel in the months and years to come? Guilt could easily destroy him, plus the fact he could end up in prison. I had to leave their house with everything crossed in the hope that he didn't go ahead with his plan.

Trying to sleep with my mind churning, revisiting the events of the day, was pointless. Questioning my actions, had I done the right thing? Was I guilty of misconduct? I could see myself in the court giving evidence! It was hell.

Selfishly, at my next visit I was willing Richard 'please be alive', over and over, just so I could have peace of mind but my heart really wanted it over for him. I opened the door, Richard was there in bed coughing and gurgling (phew)! Inwardly I breathed a sigh of relief. The feeding regime continued despite our protestations. My manager stated that she agreed with us but there was nothing she could do to change things. I despaired, it was inhumane in my opinion.

On the whole, end of life care has been an absolute joy for me. Weird statement I know, but it's true. It's such an honor to be able to help at such a crucial time. In this case however it was terrible. Richard had three weeks of hell before he could leave.

Together with A, my colleague, we set about reloading the drugs in the syringe driver. Suddenly, Richard expelled what felt like a bucket of mucous and green secretions from his nose, mouth and even his eyes. It was shocking. Then, gradually his breathing slowed and stopped. Roxanne, A and myself were the only people present. Our emotions poured out with relief. At last it was over.

It took us half an hour to feel that we might be able to focus on the jobs in hand. Just as we started the preparations, the doorbell rang. I answered the door, it was a friend enquiring after Richard, as she had just sensed him sitting in the passenger seat of her car. He was saying that a horse in the 4.30 at Goodwood (or something like that) was a cert for a bet. What the ****?

Mouths gaping, staring at each other, we stood dumb in disbelief. We hadn't even contacted the GP, literally no one else knew. How do you make any sense of it? My understanding of that morning is of a real spiritual encounter with Richard through their friend. Roxanne, my colleague A and I, all witnessed this.

We felt that Richard was still around us, making sure that we put that bet on. Roxanne just had to do it, one last time. Laughing and crying simultaneously, we watched as the horse limped past the finish line. It was Richards's last prank.

So many thoughts and feelings arise, when I remember our experience. Moral dilemmas like this happen in health care, more often in hospitals than in the community, mainly because the ability of modern medicine has advanced so much. Life must be preserved, regardless of the person's quality of life, I sometimes feel. Inserting a feeding tube in a person who has a terminal illness, is fine and I understand why they're useful, if you choose to try and live a little longer. (Stephen Hawking is a great example). The bit that needs sorting out, is the complication it can cause in the terminal phase. An honest discussion around these issues, should, in my opinion, be had before a doctor inserts one, at a time when the person is alert and cohesive and can make an informed choice.

We have the choice to refuse resuscitation, medical interventions, treatment, whatever, because that is the person's right. However, without the full and correct information around artificial feeding, how can a person foresee the difficulties it can bring? Or make the right choice? I had never experienced this before Richard, but I did in the following years and I raised my concerns with the appropriate person at the time, to try and prevent a repeat situation.

Roxanne and I truly believed, that in the final few weeks of his life, if Richard could have communicated, he would have shouted STOP. My only hope is that no one - patient, family, friend or nurse, ever has to go through that again.

From the spiritual part of this story, Roxanne, A and I believe that we witnessed a true event. It was impossible to feel anything but. I can't explain how or why it happened, it just did. It is mysterious and odd and that's why these types of encounter are frequently pooh poohed by many. I am 100% sure the spiritual world exists and no one will change my mind.

****

Afterthoughts

I've been pleasantly surprised by how much I've remembered, as I didn't keep a written record at the time that these events happened. Once in the zone though, it all came flooding back. A daily challenge to write even just a few lines, was easily achieved thanks to the COVID 19 lock down and my Christmas gift of an iPad.

It never felt like a chore. Writing a book, which is of a standard to be read and enjoyed (hopefully) by others, was a great achievement for me, as I didn't pay enough attention in English when I was a kid. One big tick on my bucket list!

Understanding human beings, especially in times of crisis and challenges, has given me a knowledge and a kind of wisdom, which I'm very grateful for. I love watching people and find each person's individual quirks and coping mechanisms, almost like a psychological encyclopaedia. Where does humour and strength come from? It's fascinating.

My job over the years, has been wonderful. Some of that is down to the fantastic teams of colleagues that I've been a part of. Mostly though, it's because I've had the good fortune to meet and work with some very special people. Every patient encounter was new and unique.

Yes, I had days when my patience was frayed, my stress level was unhealthily high, but thankfully they were relatively few. I also know that I pushed some of my managers to their limits but I was sensitive and compassionate about providing an excellent service and they understood that. Feeling the changes to community nursing as the focus centred on the business and efficiency model wasn't easy.

Looking back, I accept my inabilities, of which there were many. Sometimes life doesn't happen as you would like it. I remember one time, I applied for District Nurse training to degree level. The disappointment when I discovered that I was unsuccessful was immense. It spurred me on though and I managed a 2:1 BA Hons in Health Care a few years later. My greatest academic achievement.

Some people are meant to be managers but I wasn't. If I'd got the promotion I would have spent less time with patients and so had a less fulfilling career. Nursing people, rolling up my sleeves and helping them when they had greatest need was my job and I loved it.

I am very fortunate to have experienced several spiritual events both professionally and personally. I don't pretend to understand them but my mind is open and aware to what may be. It is my hope that in reading this book your views might be broadened too.

****

Acknowledgements

Firstly, I'd like to thank my patients and their families who have given me some exceptional human to human experiences over the years. By studying their behaviours I learned so much more than what is written in any nurse's manual.

My colleagues, be they nurses, doctors, receptionists, physios, the list is endless, have my sincerest gratitude and sympathy for putting up with me. I know I was a pain in the backside especially in my final years. You are all stars. You are very special people.

For proof reading and general hints and tips, Helen Dickie gave her time and valuable knowledge free of charge in remembrance of her father. Thank you.

My dearest and oldest friend Elaine. You have been so generous in sharing your knowledge and experience in writing but most of all in giving your love and encouragement. I thank you.

Finally I have to mention Paul, my husband. He has been there for me while writing this book with love, support. He is my technical guy when I get in a pickle (which is quite often). Paul has listened over the decades, when I came home from a particularly tricky day. He knew when to run the bath and leave me alone to cry it out of my system. He deserves a medal! I am so thankful to you.

****

Printed in Great Britain
by Amazon